ATRIAL FIBRILLATION

How to Maintain a Balanced and Healthy Lifestyle While Living with Atrial Fibrillation: Some Practical Tips

CARL JUAN

Table of Contents

Introductory

In atrial fibrillation (AFib), the two upper chambers of the heart (the atria) experience irregular and frequently fast electrical impulses. In atrial fibrillation (AFib), the atria fibrillate, or quiver, instead of contracting in a coordinated and rhythmic manner.

• AFib occurs when the heart's normal electrical conduction is disrupted, causing atrial contractions to occur at abnormal times. Symptoms like palpitations, shortness of breath, weariness, and dizziness can come from a heart rate that is too rapid or too slow.

Because the abnormal heart rhythm can trigger the production of blood clots in the atria, which can then migrate to other regions of the body, including the brain, AFib is associated with an increased risk of consequences, notably stroke. Therefore, people with AFib typically need medical treatment and management to regulate their heart rate, keep it in a regular rhythm, and lessen the likelihood of problems.

CHAPTER ONE
The Value of Prompt Diagnosis

Several factors make early diagnosis of atrial fibrillation (AFib) critically important to a person's health and well-being. Some of the most compelling arguments in favor of finding AFib early on are as follows:

1. Preventing Stroke: Atrial Fibrillation is a Major Risk Factor. Failure of the atria to contract normally increases the risk of blood clot formation. A stroke can be caused by a blood clot that breaks off and makes its way to the brain. Stroke risk can be greatly reduced with timely identification of AFib so that suitable therapies, such as blood-thinning drugs, can be implemented.

2. Palpitations, chest pain, dizziness, and weariness are common symptoms of atrial fibrillation and must be treated. The earlier these symptoms are recognized, the sooner the right treatments can be started to alleviate them and boost the patient's quality of life.

3. Preventing cardiac-Related Complications Untreated atrial fibrillation (AFib) can progress to more serious cardiac problems like

heart failure. These problems and cardiac stress can be avoided or lessened via early detection and treatment of AFib.

4. Individualized Care: Different forms, degrees, and causes of atrial fibrillation require different approaches to treatment. When patients are diagnosed early on, doctors can tailor their care to meet their individual requirements.

5. Treatment success can be evaluated and course corrections made based on the results of regular monitoring of patients with atrial fibrillation. The problem can be better controlled if followed up on and monitored often, which is made easier by early discovery.

6. Reducing alcohol intake and learning to cope with stress are just two examples of the kinds of lifestyle adjustments that may be helpful for people with atrial fibrillation. The ability to make these changes and boost one's general health is made possible by early detection.

7. Better Outcomes: The incidence and severity of problems from AFib decrease when the condition is diagnosed and treated early. It has the potential to improve people's health and extend their lifespans.

8. Emotional and mental health Struggling to cope with symptoms of an undetected heart ailment can be extremely trying. Early diagnosis brings relief and understanding, allowing patients to take control of their health and get the help they need.

9. Cost Savings Potential emergency room visits, hospitalizations, and long-term problems linked with AFib can be avoided if the condition is diagnosed and treated early.

Symptoms of AFib are not always present, and some people with the condition may experience no symptoms at all. Checkups, routine electrocardiograms (ECGs or EKGs), and risk factor monitoring can help discover AFib early, even in people who are unaware they have it. Talk to your doctor about your concerns about your heart health and be checked out if you have any risk factors for atrial fibrillation. Managing AFib and lowering the risks associated with it can make a huge difference if detected early.

The Heart: Its Structure and Functions

The heart is a muscular organ that pumps blood throughout the body, delivering oxygen and nutrition to the cells, tissues, and organs that need them. Its well-organized structure and four separate chambers allow for rapid blood pumping. Here is a rundown of the heart's anatomy and how it works:

1. All Chambered Up

• Atria The left atrium and the right atrium are the two upper chambers of the heart. The right atrium receives blood from the body that has been depleted of oxygen while the left atrial receives blood that has been oxygenated by the lungs.

The heart also contains two bottom chambers called ventricles (left and right). Both the left ventricle and the right ventricle are responsible for delivering blood to the body and the lungs, respectively.

2. The heart's four valves regulate the direction of blood flow inside the heart's chambers.

• The right atrium and ventricle are connected by a valve called the tricuspid valve.

• To clarify, the Mitral (Bicuspid) Valve is located between the left atrium and left ventricle.

• The right ventricle and the pulmonary artery that supplies the lungs are physically separated by a valve called the pulmonary valve.

- **Aortic Valve:** Separates the left ventricle from the aorta, which carries blood to the rest of the body.

3. The coronary arteries are a set of arteries that originate in the aorta and feed blood to the heart muscle (myocardium) with oxygen and nutrients.

How the Heart Works:

1. Vessels and Blood:

- The superior and inferior vena cava carry deoxygenated blood back to the right atrium from the rest of the body.

• As the right atrium squeezes, the tricuspid valve opens and blood flows into the right ventricle.

Blood is pumped to the lungs via the pulmonary artery after being squeezed by the right ventricle.

• The lungs are responsible for the exchange of oxygen and carbon dioxide in the blood.

• The pulmonary veins transport oxygen-rich blood back to the left atrium.

As the left atrium squeezes, the mitral valve opens and blood flows into the left ventricle.

When the heart beats, the left ventricle squeezes, forcing oxygen-rich blood through the aortic valve and into the aorta.

2. Circulatory System:

• Systole (heart contraction) and diastole (heart relaxation) are two stages of the cardiac cycle.

Blood is pushed forward during systole as the atrium and ventricle contract in unison.

• During diastole, the four chambers relax and refill with blood.

3. Transmission of Electricity:

• Controlling the heart's rhythm and ensuring coordinated contractions is the job of the heart's electrical conduction system, which consists of the SA (sinoatrial) node and AV (atrioventricular) node.

• Electrical impulses start in the SA node and contract the atria as they move through the body.

• In order to give the ventricles enough time to fill, the AV node delays the impulses.

The ventricles contract and pump blood in response to the electrical impulses that go through them.

The optimal functioning of the body's tissues depends on a steady supply of oxygenated blood, which can only be achieved through the heart's effective structure and function. Problems in the heart's structure or function can be caused by a number of different factors.

CHAPTER TWO
Heart Function and Atrial Fibrillation

There are many ways in which atrial fibrillation (AFib) can negatively impact heart function and cardiovascular health.

• In atrial fibrillation (AFib), the two top chambers of the heart (the atria) fibrillate instead of contracting normally, causing an irregular heartbeat. An irregular heartbeat is the outcome of electrical activity that is erratic and disorganized. An irregular heartbeat can result when the atria contract quickly and erratically, rather than in a coordinated fashion followed by the ventricles.

• Blood is not being pushed properly into the ventricles because the atria are not contracting regularly and efficiently. The atria may get enlarged as a result of the pooled blood.

• Many persons with AFib also suffer with tachycardia, a disease in which the heart rate is elevated above the typical resting rate. This might cause the heart to work harder, resulting in palpitations.

• The heart's capacity to pump blood to the rest of the body is hampered by the uneven beat and decreased efficiency. This can result in decreased cardiac output, which means less blood is being delivered to essential organs and tissues.

• One of the major hazards of atrial fibrillation is the development of blood clots in the atria. Blood clots can form in the fluttering atriums. Once released, these clots can move throughout the body, potentially blocking up other, equally important blood veins. The most dangerous outcome is a stroke when a clot reaches the brain.

• Complications of AFib include an increased risk of heart failure and other cardiac problems. Weakening of cardiac muscle and lower pumping capacity can result from the irregular rhythm and decreased efficiency.

• Palpitations, shortness of breath, chest pain, dizziness, and exhaustion are just some of the symptoms of atrial fibrillation that can interfere with a person's everyday life and reduce their quality of life.

• Living with AFib, particularly if symptoms are severe, can have a negative effect on a person's mental health. The instability of the illness can be quite upsetting.

• Because of the abnormal heart rhythm and related symptoms, people with AFib may find it difficult to participate in physical activities, which can have negative effects on their fitness and health.

The symptoms of AFib and the damage it does to the heart can be managed in a number of ways. Medication to regulate heart rate or keep it regular, blood-thinning drugs to prevent blood clots, cardioversion to restore normal rhythm, catheter ablation to interrupt abnormal electrical pathways in heart, and in rare cases, open heart surgery are all examples of such interventions.

Patients with AFib should collaborate closely with their healthcare teams to create an individualized treatment plan and routinely check their progress. Patients with AFib can benefit from better heart function, less symptoms, and a reduced risk of consequences like stroke with the right kind of therapy.

Atrial fibrillation: Possible Roots and Triggers

Many different things can set off episodes of atrial fibrillation (AFib). However, there are numerous common characteristics that are related with the development and worsening of AFib, even if the actual etiology of AFib in some patients may remain unknown (referred to as "idiopathic" AFib). Among these are the following:

1. AFib is more prevalent in the elderly and the risk rises with age.

2. AFib can be exacerbated by preexisting heart problems. It's possible that these things include:

- High blood pressure (hypertension).

- Ischemic heart disease

Diseases of the heart valves, including mitral valve prolapse

• Heart failure with congestion

• A disorder affecting the heart muscle known as cardiomyopathy.

• History of cardiac disease or surgery

3. AFib risk is also increased by a number of other medical problems, including:

Hyperthyroidism-related thyroid conditions.

• Lung conditions that worsen over time, such as COPD.

• Diabetes

• Overweight and obesity

4. Factors Relating to Daily Life Unhealthy lifestyle choices and practices, such as those involving:

• Drinking too much booze

Tobacco Use

• Caffeine consumption (excessive caffeine may cause AFib in some people).

• Extreme states of nervousness or stress

• Use of drugs, especially stimulants

5. A history of atrial fibrillation in one's family may indicate a hereditary predisposition to the condition.

6. Congenital or Acquired Heart Structural Abnormalities Congenital or acquired heart structural abnormalities can increase the risk of developing AFib.

7. Many different acute factors, including but not limited to:

• Infections, most notably those of the respiratory system

• Medical/Surgical Interventions

• Binge drinking over a short time frame (also known as "holiday heart syndrome").

Flu or other sudden illness

Extreme Effort o Physical Activity

8. Some drugs or chemicals may precipitate atrial fibrillation in those who are genetically predisposed.

Amphetamines and other stimulants

• Medications for asthma and other breathing disorders

• Medications used to treat irregular heartbeats (unfortunately, some meds might trigger AFib in some people)

Overuse of OTC drugs, especially decongestants

9. Inadequate amounts of potassium, magnesium, or calcium in the blood can affect the electrical activity of the heart, which can lead to arrhythmia.

Not everyone who has one of these risk factors will go on to develop AFib, and some people may experience AFib for no apparent reason at all. Furthermore, AFib can either be paroxysmal (episodic) or permanent, and the causes of episodes can differ from person to person.

Managing AFib often entails diagnosing and addressing the underlying causes, managing risk factors, and applying suitable treatment measures to control symptoms and limit the risk of consequences, such as stroke. Seek medical advice and examination if you experience symptoms of AFib or other cardiac problems to identify the best course of action for diagnosis and treatment.

CHAPTER THREE
The Signs and the Scrutiny

There is a wide variety of symptoms that can accompany atrial fibrillation (AFib), however it is crucial to remember that some people with AFib may have no symptoms at all. The severity of the following symptoms is variable and may be present when symptoms do occur:

- **Palpitations:** A noticeable, irregular, or fast heartbeat, typically characterized as a fluttering or pounding sensation in the chest.

• Tiredness or lack of energy that persists despite enough rest is called fatigue.

• Breathing difficulties or an overwhelming feeling of being out of breath, typically while exercising.

• Although less prevalent than other symptoms, chest pain or discomfort may be experienced by some people with AFib.

• Lightheadedness or dizziness may develop, especially upon rapidly rising to an upright position.

• **Syncope (Fainting):** AFib has been linked to a sudden loss of consciousness, or syncope, in some patients, most typically due to a drop in blood pressure.

• Anxiety The abnormal heartbeat and its symptoms might cause anxious feelings.

• To be physically weak or to notice a decline in one's physical abilities is to experience weakness.

Several procedures are frequently used in AFib diagnosis, including:

• Symptoms, risk factors, and family history of AFib and other heart diseases will all be carefully documented by a healthcare provider as part of a thorough medical history.

• **Physical Examination:** A physical examination may uncover indicators such as an irregular pulse, abnormal heart sounds, or other cardiac abnormalities.

• AFib is typically diagnosed by an electrocardiogram (ECG or EKG). It monitors the heart's electrical activity and detects arrhythmias.

• People with sporadic or paroxysmal AFib may benefit from using a Holter monitor to track their heart rate and rhythm. This portable device monitors the heart's electrical activity over an extended period of time (often 24 hours but sometimes longer).

• A device similar to a Holter monitor, an event monitor records electrical heart activity only when symptoms are present. Its typical duration of use is several hours.

• Thyroid problems and electrolyte imbalances, both of which have been linked to AFib, can be ruled out with a blood test.

• An echocardiogram is a type of ultrasonic imaging that shows the heart's structure and function in great detail. The size and function of the heart's chambers can be evaluated, and underlying structural abnormalities can be detected.

• In order to determine how your heart reacts to exercise or stress, your doctor may recommend a stress test.

• Additional Imaging Tests: Additional imaging tests, such as a chest X-ray or cardiac magnetic resonance imaging (MRI), may be utilized to evaluate lung and heart health if necessary.

medicine to control heart rate or maintain normal rhythm, blood-thinning medicine to lower the risk of blood clots and stroke, and changes to one's lifestyle may all be part of the treatment plan once atrial fibrillation (AFib) has been diagnosed. The goals of treatment are symptom management, complication avoidance, and enhanced cardiovascular health.

If you suspect you have AFib or are experiencing symptoms, it's vital to seek medical assessment and diagnosis, as early discovery and adequate care can dramatically improve results and reduce the risk of complications.

Atrial fibrillation: Classification and Types

The length and persistence of atrial fibrillation (AFib) are used to define its various subtypes. The proper approach and management to treating AFib can be determined by its classification, which is why it is so useful to doctors. AFib can be broken down into the following broad categories:

1. Infrequent or Spasmodic Atrial Fibrillation:

• Paroxysmal AFib is characterized by bouts of AFib that start unexpectedly and subsequently stop on their own, often within seven days or commonly in less than 24 hours.

Paroxysmal atrial fibrillation (AFib) is characterized by irregular and brief episodes of an abnormal heart rhythm followed by a spontaneous restoration to a normal sinus rhythm.

2. Atrial fibrillation that won't go away:

• AFib that persists for longer than seven days and does not resolve on its own is considered persistent.

• Medication or electrical cardioversion (a regulated electric shock) may be used to restore normal cardiac rhythm in patients with chronic AFib.

3. Atrial fibrillation that lasts a long time despite treatment:

• When AFib lasts longer than a year, we call it "long-standing persistent AFib," a subtype of persistent AFib.

• Catheter ablation and other ablative therapies may be considered for patients with long-standing chronic AFib who have not achieved sinus rhythm after medical therapy.

4. Atrial fibrillation that won't go away:

• When AFib lasts for an extended period of time and is either irreversible or not treatable, it is categorized as permanent AFib.

• In cases of permanent AFib, healthcare providers and patients may decide that sustaining AFib, but treating it with drugs and other therapy, is the most suitable course of action.

Note that a person's classification of AFib may alter over time depending on factors such as the frequency, duration, and responsiveness to treatment. The therapy and management of symptoms associated with AFib may also differ based on the type of AFib the patient has.

The purpose of treating atrial fibrillation is to restore normal heart rhythm, slow the heart rate, and lessen the likelihood of consequences, most notably stroke. Medication to regulate heart rate and rhythm, blood-thinning drugs to prevent blood clots, and surgical treatments such as cardioversion (restoring a normal rhythm with electrical shock) and catheter ablation (fixing faulty electrical circuits in the heart) may all be used to treat arrhythmias.

Patients with AFib should collaborate closely with their doctors to develop a treatment strategy that takes into account their unique condition and health requirements. Treatment efficacy can only be gauged and course corrections made with consistent monitoring and follow-up.

CHAPTER FOUR
Therapeutics and Administration

Strategies to regulate heart rate, keep a normal rhythm, and lessen the likelihood of consequences, most notably stroke, are central to the treatment and management of atrial fibrillation (AFib). Different types and degrees of AFib, as well as individual patient characteristics, can necessitate different approaches to treatment and care. Common methods and treatments for atrial fibrillation include as follows:

1. Managed Pricing:

• Since people with AFib frequently experience rapid contractions of the atria, rate control works to calm down the heart rate. Common medications used for this purpose include beta-blockers, calcium channel blockers, and digoxin.

• Lowering your heart rate can help alleviate some of your symptoms, cut down on the oxygen your heart needs, and make it work better overall.

2. Tempo Regulation:

• Sinus rhythm, in which the heart beats regularly, is the goal of rhythm control. Medication or surgical techniques like cardioversion can do this.

• Medication such as amiodarone, flecainide, or propafenone, known as antiarrhythmics, may be provided to assist keep the heart beating at a regular rate.

To restore a normal cardiac rhythm, cardioversion uses an electrical shock to the heart.

3. Blood-Thinning Medications (Anticoagulants):

• People with AFib are more likely to develop blood clots, which can result in a stroke. Medications that thin the blood, called anticoagulants, are commonly administered to lower this danger.

• Commonly used anticoagulants include warfarin, direct oral anticoagulants (DOACs) such apixaban, dabigatran, edoxaban, and rivaroxaban.

Age, stroke risk, and bleeding risk are just a few of the characteristics that play a role in deciding which anticoagulant to use and how much to take.

4. Ablation Catheter:

• AFib can be treated with catheter ablation, a minimally invasive treatment that blocks off the faulty electrical channels in the heart.

• During the surgery, narrow catheters are introduced into the heart, and scars or lesions are created in the heart tissue using radiofrequency or cryoablation radiation to block the aberrant electrical signals.

• Patients with symptomatic AFib who do not react effectively to medicines or who prefer a non-pharmacological therapy may be candidates for catheter ablation.

5. Ablation Surgery: Surgical ablation is often reserved for patients undergoing other cardiac procedures, such as heart valve repair or bypass surgery, and is conducted during an open-heart operation.

• Lesions are made in the heart to block the conduction of erroneous electrical impulses.

6. Adjustments to Your Way of Life:

• Modifying one's way of life can be helpful in the management of AFib and the alleviation of symptoms. It's possible that these things include:

Reducing one's alcohol intake

Reducing Anxiety

• The importance of reaching and keeping a healthy weight

Practicing frequent physical activity, as suggested by a medical professional

Quitting Smoking

Taking care of preexisting illnesses like high blood pressure and diabetes

7. Checking in and Keeping Tabs:

• In order to gauge the efficacy of treatment and make any required adjustments, regular monitoring is mandatory.

ECGs, Holter monitors, and event monitors are all possible options for long-term monitoring of cardiac activity.

A patient's overall health, the type of AFib they have, and the presence of any underlying cardiac diseases all play a role in determining the best course of treatment. Together with their doctors, patients should weigh the pros and cons of available treatments to determine the best course of action. When AFib is well managed, it can improve quality of life and lessen the likelihood of problems.

Risk Factors and Adverse Events

Atrial fibrillation (AFib) is connected with numerous consequences and risk factors. For effective management and prevention of AFib, knowledge of these factors is crucial. Risk risks and potential problems are outlined below.

Complications:

• The increased risk of stroke is one of the most serious consequences of atrial fibrillation. In atrial fibrillation, blood might clot in the fluttering atrium. Stroke is caused when one of these clots breaks loose and travels to the brain.

• In the long run, AFib can cause heart failure by reducing the strength of the heart muscle. Inadequate blood pumping as a result of the heart's irregular rhythm and decreased efficiency can cause symptoms such as shortness of breath, exhaustion, and fluid retention.

• Heart Attacks and other cardiovascular events (such pulmonary emboli) are more likely to occur in people with AFib, such as when blood clots form in the veins and spread to other regions of the body.

• Palpitations, dizziness, exhaustion, and shortness of breath are just few of the symptoms of atrial fibrillation that can significantly reduce a person's quality of life.

• Due to the increased risk of stroke and decreased cerebral blood flow, AFib has been linked in certain studies to cognitive impairment or dementia.

• Anticoagulant medicines, commonly administered to individuals with atrial fibrillation in an effort to lower their stroke risk, have been linked to an increased risk of bleeding. Controlling this danger is crucial.

• Recurrent hospitalizations are a common consequence of atrial fibrillation, especially in the presence of severe symptoms or complications.

Causal Variables:

• AFib is more prevalent in the elderly and the risk rises with age.

• Hypertension, coronary artery disease, valvular heart disease, heart failure, and congenital heart defects are all underlying heart diseases that might raise the risk of AFib.

• Hypertension is a major risk factor for atrial fibrillation.

• AFib is more common in people who also have diabetes.

• Excessive fat storage can play a role in the onset of atrial fibrillation (AFib), especially when combined with other cardiovascular risk factors.

• Hyperthyroidism, often known as an overactive thyroid, has been linked to an increased risk of atrial fibrillation.

- **Lifestyle Factors**: Certain lifestyle choices and practices can raise the risk of AFib, including excessive alcohol use, smoking, and excessive caffeine intake.

- There may be a genetic susceptibility to atrial fibrillation if it runs in the family.

- Congenital or acquired structural cardiac abnormalities raise the risk of atrial fibrillation.

- **Other Medical problems**: Sleep apnea, chronic renal illness, and chronic lung disease are all problems that can increase a person's risk of developing atrial fibrillation.

Both healthcare providers and people at risk for or diagnosed with AFib need a thorough understanding of these consequences and risk factors. The risk of complications and the quality of life for people with AFib can be reduced and enhanced, respectively, through the identification and treatment of modifiable risk factors. Treatment, lifestyle changes, and routine medical checkups are all crucial for keeping AFib under control.

CHAPTER FIVE
Managing Atrial Fibrillation in Daily Life

Atrial fibrillation (AFib) is a cardiac rhythm disorder that requires vigilant management and behavioral changes to keep the heart healthy and lessen the likelihood of consequences. Some important things to keep in mind if you have AFib:

1. Medical Management: If your doctor has prescribed medicine to lower your blood pressure, stabilize your heart rate, or prevent blood clots, take them exactly as directed. Be careful to keep any follow-up appointments with your doctor and take any prescribed drugs as advised.

2. Take anticoagulants (blood thinners) as recommended if your doctor has told you to do so to lower your risk of stroke. Know the potential side effects of these drugs and talk about your worries with your doctor.

3. Adjustments to Your Way of Life:

• Fruits, vegetables, whole grains, lean proteins, and a diet low in saturated and trans fats are all part of a heart-healthy diet. To control blood pressure, a low-sodium diet is recommended.

• Follow your doctor's orders and make exercise a consistent part of your routine. Regular exercise has been shown to enhance cardiovascular health and reduce AFib symptoms.

• Caffeine and alcohol should be consumed in moderation, as both can set off AFib in some people. Caffeine might affect your heart rate, so use caution if you often consume it.

The symptoms of atrial fibrillation (AFib) can be made worse by stress, so it's important to learn stress-reduction practices like deep breathing, meditation, or yoga.

When it comes to your heart's health, nothing is more important than giving up smoking. When it comes to AFib, smoking is a huge red flag.

4. Track Your Signs: Keep tabs on how you're feeling and let your doctor know right away if anything seems off. Document the dates, times, and severity of your AFib episodes in a diary.

5. Blood Pressure Control: If you have hypertension, cooperate with your healthcare professional to manage and control your blood pressure properly.

6. Don't let yourself get dehydrated; it's been linked to AFib's development and worsening. Ensure you stay well-hydrated, especially during hot weather or when indulging in vigorous exercise.

7. Consistent check-ins with your doctor are essential for keeping tabs on how well your AFib treatment is working. During these checkups, doctors can modify dosages, keep an eye on patients, and address any worries they may have.

8. Determine your personal risk of stroke and talk to your doctor about whether or not anticoagulant medication is necessary and, if so, which kind would be best for you.

9. Get informed about atrial fibrillation (AFib), its causes, and available treatments. The more you understand about your illness, the more actively you can participate in your care, and the better decisions you can make for yourself.

10. Know when to seek medical assistance or phone 911 in the event of serious symptoms, especially if they are new or more severe than usual.

11. You may want to look into AFib-specific support groups or study up on the topic on your own. Connecting with people who have AFib can provide significant insights and emotional support.

12. Precautions for Traveling: If you are taking anticoagulants, you should let your doctor know about your trip plans. Make sure you know how to handle your condition while away from home and that you have enough medication to last the duration of your trip.

Keep in mind that treating AFib is a continuous process. Collaborate together with your medical staff to develop individualized plans for treatment and behavioral modifications. Many people who have AFib can live normal, active lives and lower their risk of problems with the right kind of care.

Atrial Fibrillation Prevention

Preventing atrial fibrillation (AFib) may not always be possible, especially in cases where AFib is related with underlying medical disorders or hereditary factors. However, there are a number of ways to lessen the likelihood of developing AFib or its complications, including changes to one's lifestyle and the treatment of risk factors.

1. Take Care of Preexisting Conditions: Collaborate with your doctor to maintain healthy levels of high blood pressure, diabetes, or thyroid diseases. Comorbidities can be addressed to lessen the likelihood of developing AFib.

2. Keep Your Weight Down:

• Obesity, specifically, is associated with a higher incidence of AFib. A balanced diet and regular exercise can help you keep your weight down and lower your risk.

3. Consistent Physical Activity:

• Make exercise a consistent part of your routine. Aim for at least 75 minutes of intense exercise every week, or 150 minutes of moderate exercise. Physical activity has been shown to improve cardiovascular health and lower the incidence of AFib.

4. Fruits, vegetables, whole grains, lean proteins, and healthy fats should make up the bulk of your diet, while saturated fats, trans fats, and sodium should be kept to a

minimum. The risk of cardiovascular disease and atrial fibrillation can both be lowered by following such a diet.

5. Cut back on the booze:

• Some people develop atrial fibrillation (AFib) when they drink too much alcohol. If you drink alcohol, do it in moderation. Talk to your doctor about what the word "moderate" means in the context of your health.

6. Stress Management:

• Persistent stress may exacerbate preexisting cardiac rhythm disorders. Practice stress-reduction strategies such as deep breathing, meditation, yoga, or activities you like.

7. Intake of Caffeine:

• Excessive caffeine use can bring up AFib in certain people. Be conscious of how much caffeine you're consuming and how it affects your pulse rate.

8. Do not Smoke:

• If you smoke, stopping is one of the most critical things you can do to protect your heart and lower the chance of AFib. Heart disease and atrial fibrillation both have smoking as a major risk factor.

9. Avoid dehydration:

• AFib can be brought on or made worse by dehydration. Keep yourself well hydrated, especially when it's hot out or when you're working up a sweat.

10. Even if you feel OK, it is important to keep up with your doctor's recommended checkup schedule. The onset of atrial fibrillation (AFib) can be delayed with the early identification and control of risk factors.

11. Coffee with alcohol in moderation:

• Caffeine and alcohol are generally thought to be safe for most people when used in moderation; nevertheless, excessive intake can precipitate AFib in some individuals. Think about how much you're drinking in relation to how it might affect your heart rate.

12. Medication Compliance: If you have a medical condition that requires medication, take your prescriptions as prescribed by your healthcare practitioner to manage your condition properly.

Although these interventions can lessen the likelihood of developing AFib, they may not remove it completely, especially in cases of AFib for which no reason can be determined. Talking to your doctor about your specific worries and risk factors for AFib will help them give you with tailored advice and monitoring to lower your chances of getting AFib or its complications.

Conclusion

When left untreated, atrial fibrillation (AFib) can have serious consequences for a person's cardiovascular system and overall health. In AFib, the upper chambers (atria) of the heart contract irregularly and rapidly, which can cause a variety of symptoms and raise the risk of consequences, the most serious of which is stroke.

• The ability to promptly intervene and control AFib makes early detection essential. Because it has the ability to improve heart function and quality of life for people with AFib, early identification is crucial. Managing atrial fibrillation and lowering related risks is greatly aided by early diagnosis and individualized treatment plans.

• Catheter ablation is just one of many medical treatments used in the treatment and management of atrial fibrillation (AFib), along with other methods like as rate control, rhythm control, anticoagulation (blood thinning), dietary changes, and behavioral adjustments. The goals of these approaches are symptom management, reduced risk of complications, and enhanced cardiovascular health.

It is crucial for both healthcare providers and people living with AFib to have an understanding of the difficulties and risk factors related with the condition. It is possible to lessen the likelihood of problems and boost the quality of life for persons with AFib by addressing modifiable risk factors and managing the condition appropriately.

• Maintaining regular follow-up consultations with a healthcare professional is an important part of taking an active role in managing one's health while living with AFib. With careful management and a commitment to heart-healthy choices, many patients with AFib can have satisfying lives and lower their risk of problems.

• Although it is not always possible to prevent AFib, the chance of having AFib can be decreased by adopting a heart-healthy lifestyle and controlling risk factors. The protection of cardiovascular health and general health can be greatly aided by the awareness of personal risk factors and the implementation of preventative actions.

Managing the effects of AFib and lowering the risk of complications requires aggressive care and lifestyle changes. The management and prevention of atrial fibrillation rely on early detection, effective treatment, and preventative measures.

THE END

www.ingramcontent.com/pod-product-compliance
Lightning Source LLC
Chambersburg PA
CBHW050744260726
48661CB00001B/396